翻 译/汪芳俊
执 行/曲建鹏
手法演示/舒剑锋
摄 影/王 浩

6招搞定

手到病除

范炳华 著

浙江科学技术出版社

Six STEPS TO RELIEVE SYMPTOMS

图书在版编目（CIP）数据

手到病除，6招搞定 / 范炳华著 . -- 杭州：浙江科学技术出版社，2016.8
ISBN 978-7-5341-7273-1

Ⅰ . ①手… Ⅱ . ①范… Ⅲ . ①按摩疗法（中医）－基本知识 Ⅳ . ① R244.1

中国版本图书馆 CIP 数据核字（2016）第 200189 号

书　　名	手到病除，6招搞定
英文书名	SIX STEPS TO RELIEVE SYMPTOMS
著　　者	范炳华

翻译 / 汪芳俊　　执行 / 曲建鹏　　手法演示 / 舒剑锋　　摄影 / 王浩

出版发行	浙江科学技术出版社
	杭州市体育场路 347 号　邮政编码：310006
	办公室电话：0571-85176593
	销售部电话：0571-85176040
	网　址：www.zkpress.com
	E-mail：zkpress@zkpress.com
排　　版	杭州兴邦电子印务有限公司
印　　刷	杭州下城教育印刷有限公司

开　　本	787mm × 1092mm　　1/32	印　张	3.5
字　　数	70 000		
版　　次	2016 年 8 月第 1 版	印　次	2016 年 8 月第 1 次印刷
书　　号	ISBN 978-7-5341-7273-1	定　价	28.00 元

版权所有　翻印必究
（图书出现倒装、缺页等印装质量问题，本社销售部负责调换）

责任编辑	沈秋强　刘 丹	责任校对	梁　峥
责任美编	金　晖	责任印务	田　文

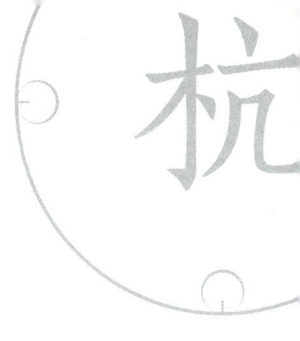

前言

推拿（按摩）是中医学的重要组成部分，有文字记载已有2000多年的历史，具有医疗、保健、养生的作用，是中华民族灿烂的文化瑰宝。

本书精选于1999年由浙江科学技术出版社出版的《中老年常见病症自我推拿保健疗法》一书，该著作曾获"浙江省科学技术进步奖三等奖"。本书节选了该书中高血压、失眠、眩晕、头痛等14个易操作、易理解、易掌握的代表性病症，以期读者朋友们能够通过自我推拿来达到医疗、养生、保健的目的。

感谢我的编写团队为此书的出版所付出的辛勤劳动，感谢浙江科学技术出版社的敬业与专业。

谨以此书献给在美丽的西子湖畔举办的G20峰会。

浙江中医药大学　范炳华

2016年7月于杭州

Preface

    Tui Na (An Mo) is an essential component of Traditional Chinese Medicine with a history of more than 2,000 years. It is a treasure in the splendid Chinese culture serving people's health and medical care.

    This booklet has been carefully selected from the *Self-massage Therapy for Common Senile Disease* published by Zhejiang Science and Technology Publishing House. This work was awarded the 3rd Prize of Zhejiang Science and Technology Progress Award.14 simple manipulations in Tui Na for the common diseases such as hypertension, insomnia, vertigo and headache were selected from the book, helping readers to understand and learn self-massage in the purpose of treatment and health care.

    Here I would like to express my gratitude to my editing group for the hard work they did for the publishing of this book, as well as the professional dedication of Zhejiang Science and Technology Publishing House.

    I would like to dedicate this book to the G20 Summit, to be held in Hangzhou, beside the beautiful West Lake.

Fan Binghua
Zhejiang Chinese Medical University
Hangzhou
July 2016

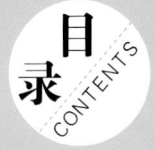

高血压 Hypertension / 2

失眠 Insomnia / 10

眩晕 Vertigo / 18

头痛 Headache / 26

慢性结肠炎 Chronic Colitis / 34

习惯性便秘 Constipation / 40

视疲劳 Eye Fatigue / 48

牙痛 Toothache / 56

颈椎病 Neck Pain / 62

腰肌劳损 Lumbar Strain / 70

肩关节周围炎 Shoulder Pain (Frozen Shoulder) / 78

增生性膝关节炎 Knee Osteoarthritis / 86

跟痛症 Heel Pain Syndrome / 94

慢性鼻炎 Chronic Rhinitis / 102

高血压
Hypertension

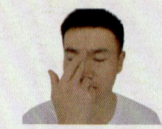

1 按揉印堂穴
Press and knead Yin Tang point

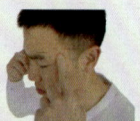

2 按揉太阳穴
Press and knead Tai Yang point

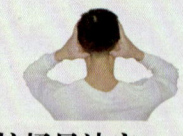

3 按揉风池穴
Press and knead Feng Chi point

4 抹降压沟
Wipe Jiang Ya Gou

5 抹桥弓
Wipe Qiao Gong

6 擦涌泉穴
Rub Yong Quan point

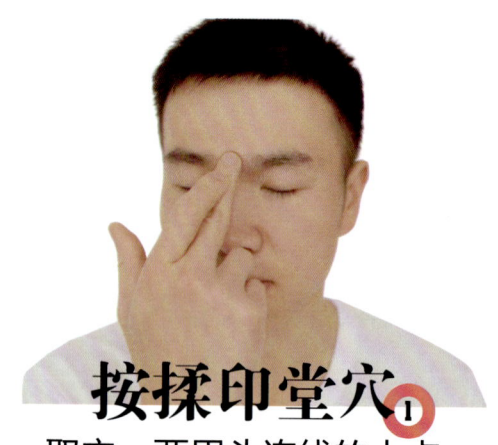

按揉印堂穴 ①
取穴：两眉头连线的中点

方法
用中指螺纹面按揉 100 次。
要领
手法用力宜轻柔，带动皮下组织按揉。

Press and knead Yin Tang point
Location
At the midpoint of the line joining the medial ends of the two eyebrows.
Manipulation
Press and knead the point with middle finger, 100 times.
Key
Press and knead the point together with the soft tissue underneath with gentle force.

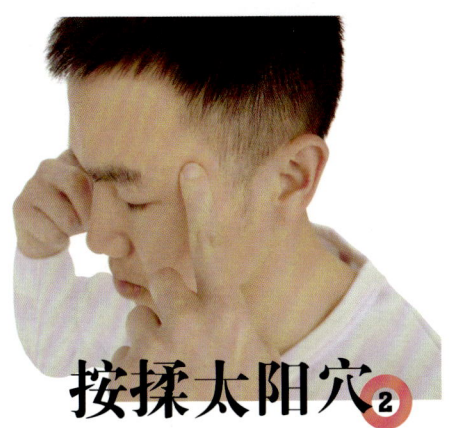

按揉太阳穴 2
取穴：眉梢与目外眦之间向后约1寸凹陷处

方法
用双手食指螺纹面同时按揉100次。
要领
操作时精神要放松，意念集中于太阳穴，手法用力宜轻柔，带动皮下组织按揉。

Press and knead Tai Yang point
Location
1 cun posterior to the eyebrow and outer canthus.
Manipulation
Press and knead the points with both index fingers, 100 times.
Key
While manipulating focus your mind on the point, press and knead the point gently together with the soft tissue underneath.

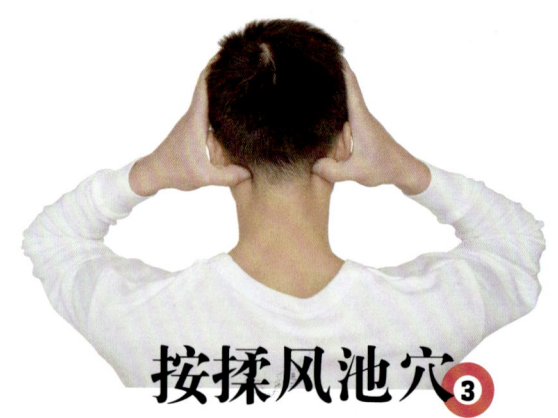

按揉风池穴 ❸

取穴：十指自然张开抱头，拇指往上推，在脖子与发际的交界线各有一凹处（风府穴与颞骨乳突之间的凹陷处）

方法
用双手拇指螺纹面同时按揉 100 次。

要领
拇指螺纹面按于风池穴紧贴枕骨上缘按揉，使局部有酸胀麻感。

Press and knead Feng Chi point

Location
Hold the back of head with ten fingers upwards,
your thumb will find a depression between the upper ends of the sternocleidomastoid and trapezius muscles.

Manipulation
Press and knead the points with both thumbs, 100 times.

Key
You will feel sore while pressing and kneading the point.

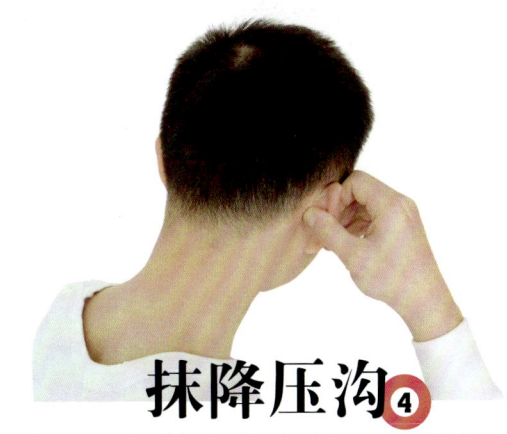

抹降压沟 ④
取穴：耳郭的内上方斜向外下方走行

方法
用拇指螺纹面沿降压沟自内上向外下推抹，左右各100次。

要领
用拇指螺纹面自耳郭背面隆起的上端向耳垂方向单方向抹动。

Wipe Jiang Ya Gou

Location

In the depression on the back of the auricle, rub downwards.

Manipulation

Wipe downwards with thumb, 100 times each side.

Key

Wipe in a single direction up to down only.

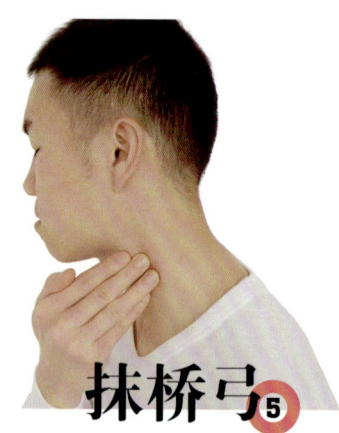

抹桥弓 ⑤

取穴：耳后翳风穴（耳垂后耳根部）至缺盆穴（锁骨上窝中央）连线

方法
用食指、中指、无名指和小指的螺纹面自上而下抹桥弓，左右各 20 次。

要领
自耳后向前下至缺盆穴单方向抹动，左手推右侧，右手推左侧。手法用力宜轻柔，频率宜稍快。

Wipe Qiao Gong

Location
Connecting the line between earlobe and supraclavicular fossa.

Manipulation
Manipulate with index, middle, ring and little fingers, 20 times each side.

Key
Wipe in a single direction from earlobe to supraclavicular fossa, with left hand for right side, right hand for left side; gently and frequently.

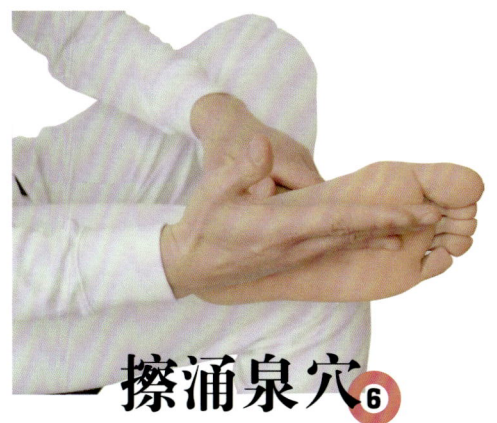

擦涌泉穴 ❻
取穴：足底前 1/3 人字缝的凹陷处

方法
用小鱼际（手掌小指侧肌肉丰满处）擦涌泉穴，左手擦右侧，
右手擦左侧，左右各 100 次，早晚各 1 次。

要领
小鱼际部着力来回摩擦，手法用力宜轻柔，频率稍快，
摩擦的距离宜稍长，足底有明显温热感。

Rub Yong Quan point
Location
In the depression $1/3^{rd}$ down and $2/3^{rd}$ up the middle line
of the sole of the foot when the foot is flexed.

Manipulation
Rub Yong Quan point with hypothenar
100 times each side, twice a day, in the morning and evening.

Key
Rub gently and frequently with hypothenar
back and forth, until it feels warm.

失眠
Insomnia

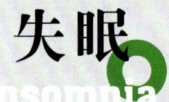

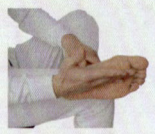
1 擦涌泉穴
Rub Yong Quan point

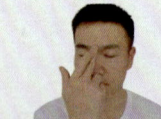
2 按揉印堂穴
Press and knead Yin Tang point

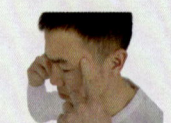
3 按揉太阳穴
Press and knead Tai Yang point

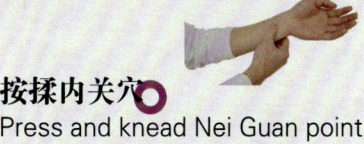

4 按揉内关穴
Press and knead Nei Guan point

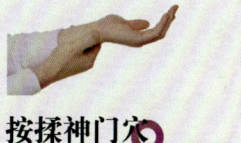

5 按揉神门穴
Press and knead Shen Men point

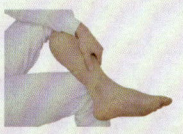

6 按揉三阴交穴
Press and knead San Yin Jiao point

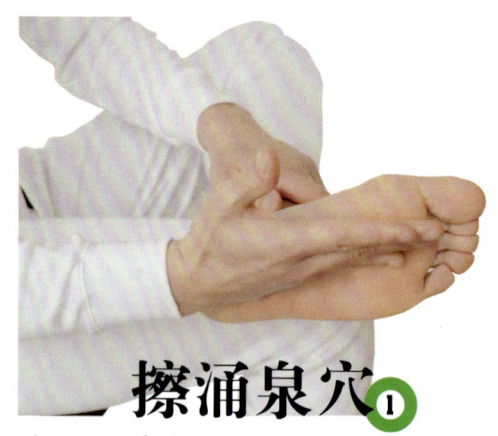

擦涌泉穴 ①
取穴：足底前 1/3 人字缝的凹陷处

方法
用小鱼际（手掌小指侧肌肉丰满处）擦涌泉穴，左手擦右侧，右手擦左侧，左右各 100 次，早晚各 1 次。

要领
双膝屈曲，一足置于对侧膝关节上，用左手擦右侧，右手擦左侧，手法用力宜轻柔，频率稍快，摩擦的距离宜稍长，使足底明显透热。

Rub Yong Quan point
Location
In the depression 1/3rd down and 2/3rd up the middle line of the sole of the foot when the foot is flexed.

Manipulation
Rub Yong Quan point with hypothenar 100 times each side, twice a day, in the morning and evening.

Key
Rub gently and frequently with hypothenar back and forth, until it feels warm.

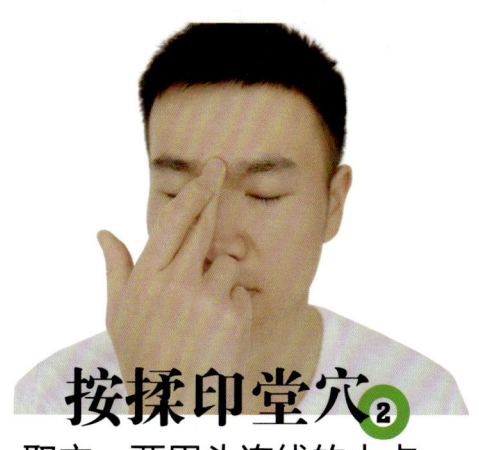

按揉印堂穴 ❷
取穴：两眉头连线的中点

方法

用中指螺纹面按揉 100 次。

要领

手法用力宜轻柔，带动皮下组织按揉，
意念集中于穴位上。

Press and knead Yin Tang point

Location

At midpoint of the connecting line
between the ends of the two eyebrows.

Manipulation

Press and knead the point with middle finger, 100 times.

Key

Press and knead the point together with the
soft tissue underneath with gentle force.

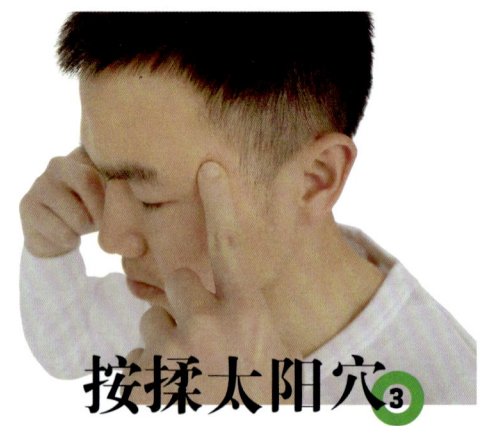

按揉太阳穴 ❸

取穴：眉梢与目外眦之间向后约 1 寸凹陷处

方法
用双手食指螺纹面同时按揉 100 次。

要领
操作时精神要放松，意念集中于太阳穴，手法用力宜轻柔，带动皮下组织按揉。

Press and knead Tai Yang point

Location

1 cun posterior to the eyebrow and outer canthus.

Manipulation

Press and knead the points with both index fingers, 100 times.

Key

Focus your mind on the point while manipulating, press and knead the point gently together with the soft tissue underneath.

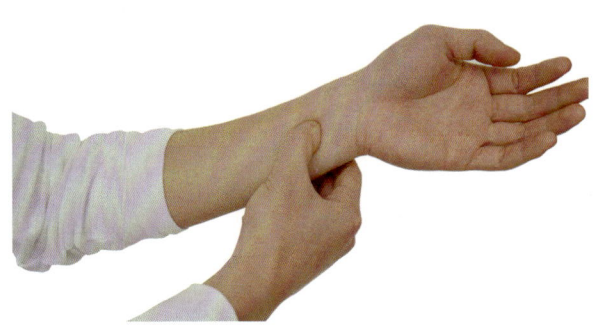

按揉内关穴 ④
取穴：前臂正中，腕横纹上 2 寸，掌长肌腱与桡侧腕屈肌腱之间

方法
用拇指螺纹面按揉，左右各 100 次。
要领
左手按揉右侧穴位，右手按揉左侧穴位，手法用力宜深沉，使局部有酸胀感。

Press and knead Nei Guan point
Location
2 cun above the transverse crease of the wrist, between the tendons of palmaris longus and flexor carpi radialis.
Manipulation
Press and knead the point with thumb, 100 times each side.
Key
Manipulate with deep strength, and make the point feel sore.

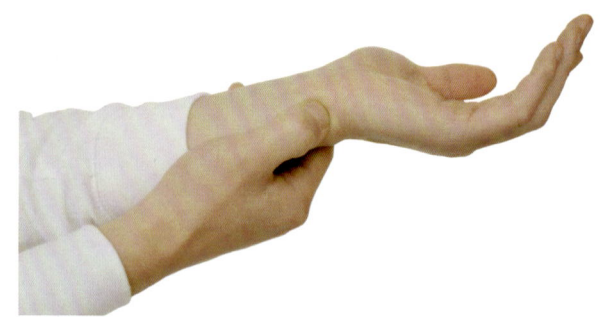

按揉神门穴 ⑤
取穴：腕横纹尺侧（小指侧）端

方法
用拇指螺纹面按揉，左右各 100 次。
要领
左手按揉右侧穴位，右手按揉左侧穴位，
手法用力宜适中，使局部有酸胀感。

Press and knead Shen Men point
Location
On the palmar, ulnar end of the transverse crease of the wrist.
Manipulation
Press and knead the point with thumb,
100 times each side.
Key
Manipulate with medium strength and make the point feel sore.

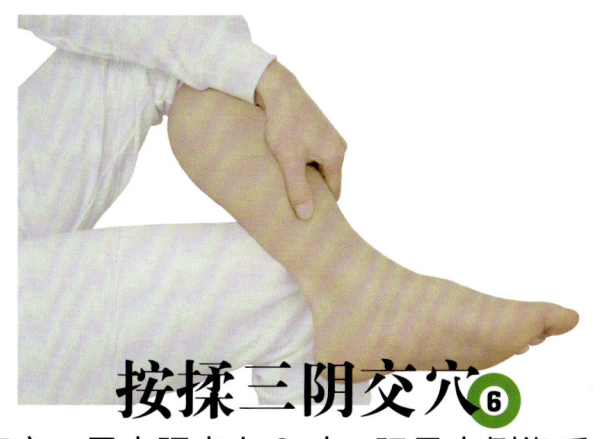

按揉三阴交穴 ❻
取穴：足内踝尖上 3 寸，胫骨内侧缘后方

方法

用拇指螺纹面按揉，左右各 100 次。

要领

拇指螺纹面紧贴胫骨内侧面，
手法用力宜适中，使局部有酸胀感。

Press and knead San Yin Jiao point

Location

3 cun above the tip of the medial malleolus
and posterior to the inner edge of the tibia.

Manipulation

Press and knead the point with thumb,
100 times each side.

Key

Manipulate with medium strength and make the point feel sore.

眩晕
Vertigo

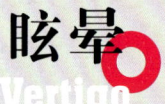

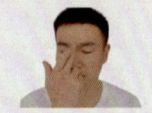

1 按揉印堂穴
Press and knead Yin Tang point

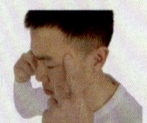

2 按揉太阳穴
Press and knead Tai Yang point

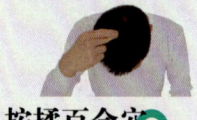

3 按揉百会穴
Press and knead Bai Hui point

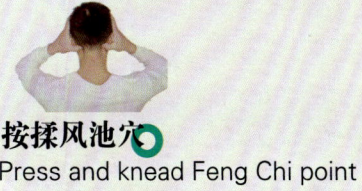

4 按揉风池穴
Press and knead Feng Chi point

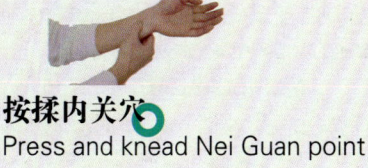

5 按揉翳风穴
Press and knead Yi Feng point

6 按揉内关穴
Press and knead Nei Guan point

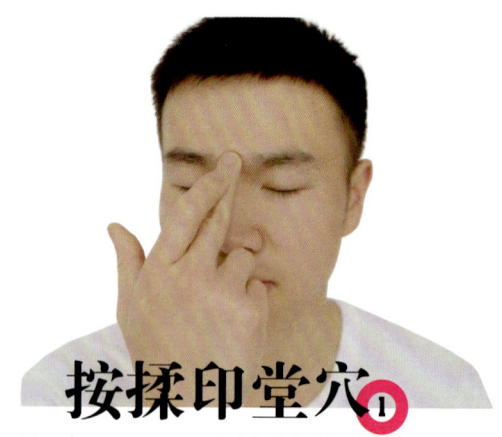

按揉印堂穴 ❶
取穴：两眉头连线的中点

方法
用中指螺纹面按揉 100 次。

要领
手法用力宜轻柔，带动皮下组织按揉，
意念集中于穴位上。

Press and knead Yin Tang point

Location
At the midpoint of the line joining the medial ends of the two eyebrows.

Manipulation
Press and knead the point with middle finger, 100 times.

Key
Focus your mind on the point while manipulating, press and knead the point gently together with the soft tissue underneath.

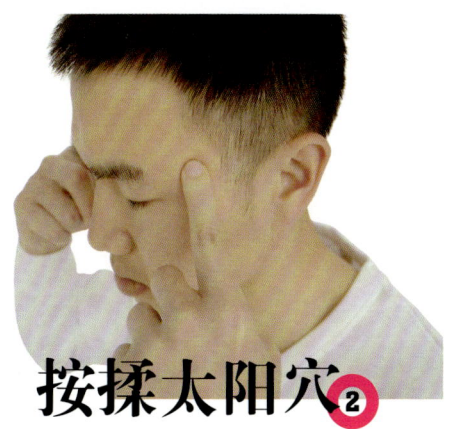

按揉太阳穴 ❷

取穴：眉梢与目外眦之间向后约 1 寸凹陷处

方法
用双手食指螺纹面同时按揉 100 次。

要领
操作时精神要放松，意念集中于太阳穴，手法用力宜轻柔，带动皮下组织按揉。

Press and knead Tai Yang point

Location

1 cun posterior to the eyebrow and outer canthus.

Manipulation

Press and knead the points with both index fingers, 100 times.

Key

Focus your mind on the point while manipulating, press and knead the point gently together with the soft tissue underneath.

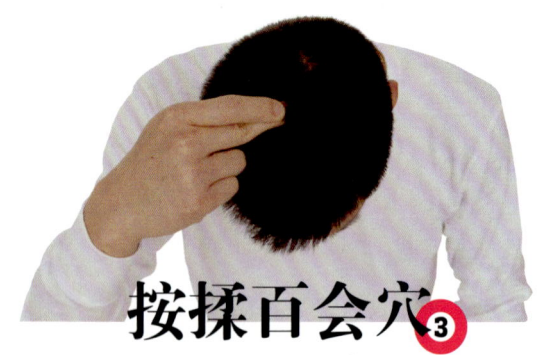

按揉百会穴 ③

取穴：两耳尖直上，
头顶与前后正中线交会处

方法

用中指螺纹面按揉 100 次。

要领

手法用力宜适中，带动皮下组织按揉，
意念集中于整个头部，使局部有轻度酸胀感。

Press and knead Bai Hui point

Location

On the middle line of the back of the head,
7 cun directly above the midpoint of the posterior hairline.

Manipulation

Press and knead the point with middle finger, 100 times.

Key

Press and knead the point together with the soft tissue underneath
with medium force, while focusing your mind on the head,
until the point feels sore.

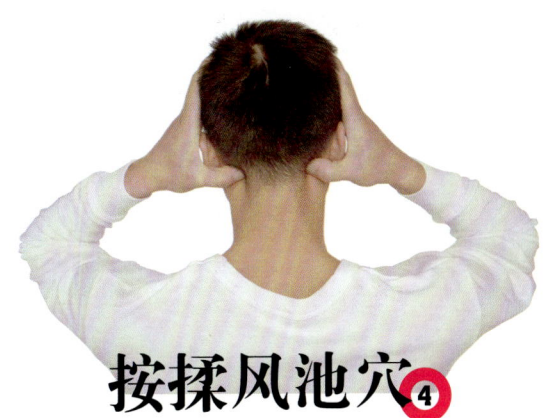

按揉风池穴 ④

取穴：十指自然张开抱头，拇指往上推，在脖子与发际的交界线各有一凹处（风府穴与颞骨乳突之间的凹陷处）

方法
用双手拇指螺纹面同时按揉 100 次。

要领
拇指螺纹面按于风池穴紧贴枕骨上缘按揉，手法用力宜适中，使局部有酸胀麻感。

Press and knead Feng Chi point

Location
Hold the back of head with ten fingers upwards,
your thumb will find a depression between the upper ends of the sternocleidomastoid and trapezius muscles.

Manipulation
Press and knead the points with both thumbs, 100 times.

Key
You will feel sore while pressing and kneading the point.

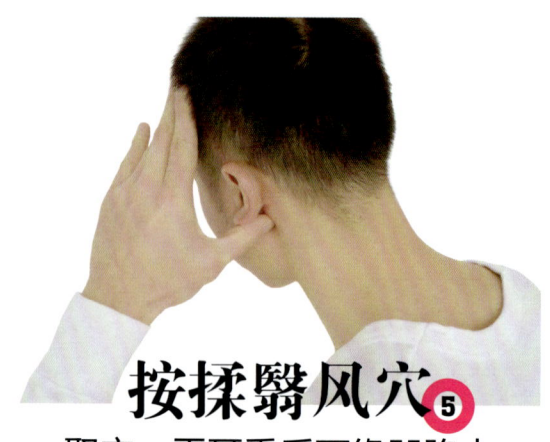

按揉翳风穴 ❺
取穴：平耳垂后下缘凹陷中

方法
用拇指指端同时按揉 100 次。

要领
两手拇指指端按于两侧穴位上，余四指扶于头部进行按揉，手法用力宜轻柔，使局部有酸胀感。

Press and knead Yi Feng point
Location
In the depression behind the earlobe.
Manipulation
Press and knead the points with both thumbs, 100 times.
Key
Press with thumb on the point while the other four fingers holding the head with gentle force.

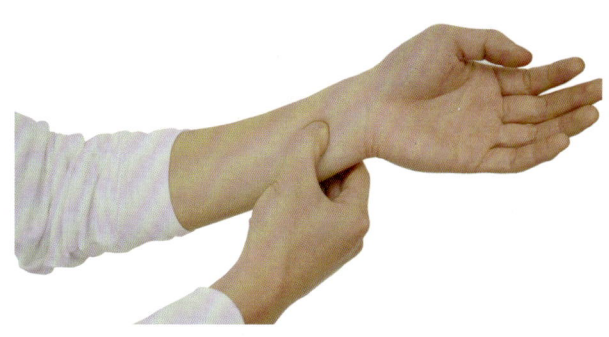

按揉内关穴 ❻
取穴：前臂正中，腕横纹上 2 寸

方法
用拇指螺纹面按揉，左右各 100 次。
要领
左手按揉右侧穴位，右手按揉左侧穴位，手法用力宜深沉，使局部有酸胀感。

Press and knead Nei Guan point
Location
2 cun above the transverse crease of the wrist.
Manipulation
Press and knead the point with thumb, 100 times each side.
Key
Press and knead the point with deep force and make it feel sore.

头痛
Headache

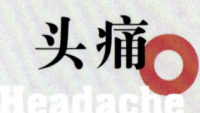

1 按揉印堂穴
Press and knead Yin Tang point

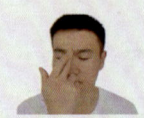

2 按揉太阳穴
Press and knead Tai Yang point

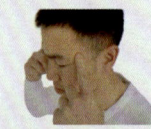

3 按揉风池穴
Press and knead Feng Chi point

4 按揉百会穴
Press and knead Bai Hui point

5 按揉率谷穴
Press and knead Shuai Gu point

6 梳理头部
Comb hair

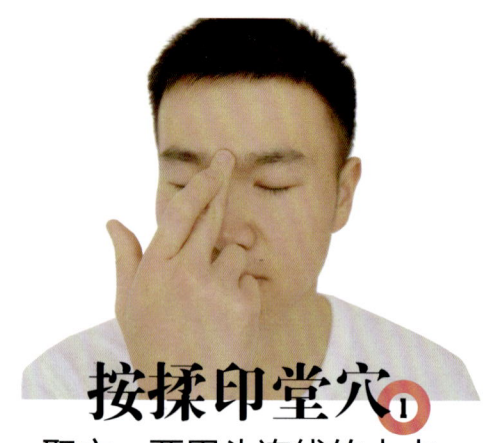

按揉印堂穴 ①
取穴：两眉头连线的中点

方法
用中指螺纹面按揉 100 次。

要领
手法用力宜轻柔，带动皮下组织按揉，意念集中于穴位上，使局部有舒适感。

Press and knead Yin Tang point

Location

At the midpoint of the line joining the medial ends of the two eyebrows.

Manipulation

Press and knead the point with middle finger, 100 times.

Key

Press and knead the point together with the soft tissue underneath with gentle force and focus your mind on the point.

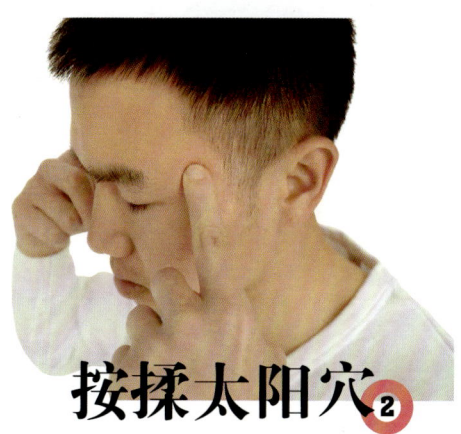

按揉太阳穴 ②
取穴：眉梢与目外眦之间向后约 1 寸凹陷处

方法
用双手食指螺纹面同时按揉 100 次。

要领
操作时精神要放松，意念集中于太阳穴，手法用力宜轻柔，带动皮下组织按揉。

Press and knead Tai Yang point

Location
1 cun posterior to the eyebrow and outer canthus.

Manipulation
Press and knead the points with both index fingers, 100 times.

Key
Focus your mind on the point while manipulating. Press and knead the point together with the soft tissue underneath gently.

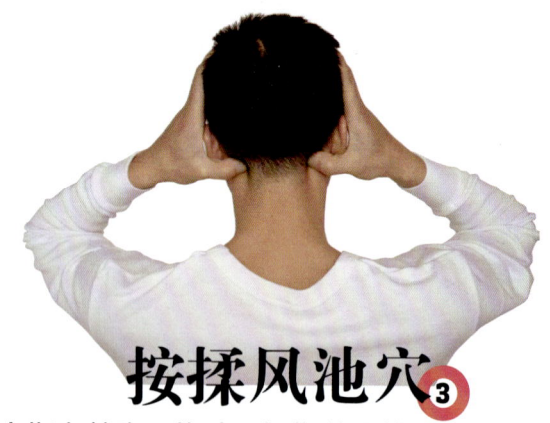

按揉风池穴 ③

取穴：十指自然张开抱头，拇指往上推，在脖子与发际的交界线各有一凹处（风府穴与颞骨乳突之间的凹陷处）

方法
用两手拇指螺纹面同时按揉 100 次。

要领
拇指螺纹面按于风池穴紧贴枕骨上缘，向内上按揉，使颞侧头部有放射样酸胀麻感。

Press and knead Feng Chi point

Location

Hold the back of head with ten fingers upwards, your thumb will find a depression between the upper ends of the sternocleidomastoid and trapezius muscles.

Manipulation

Press and knead the points with both thumbs, 100 times.

Key

Touch the upper edge of occipital bone with the thumb firmly and manipulate upwards, soreness should radiate to the temporal area.

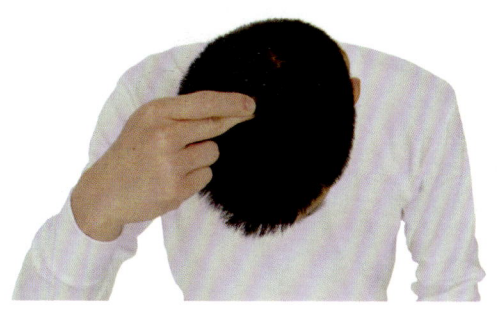

按揉百会穴 ❹
取穴：两耳尖直上，头顶与前后正中线交会处

方法
用中指螺纹面按揉 100 次。

要领
手法用力宜适中，带动皮下组织按揉，意念集中于整个头部，使局部有轻度酸胀感。

Press and knead Bai Hui point

Location

On the middle line on the back of the head, 7 cun directly above the midpoint of the posterior hairline.

Manipulation

Press and knead the point with middle finger, 100 times.

Key

Press and knead the point together with the soft tissue underneath with medium force, while focusing your mind on the head, until the point feels sore.

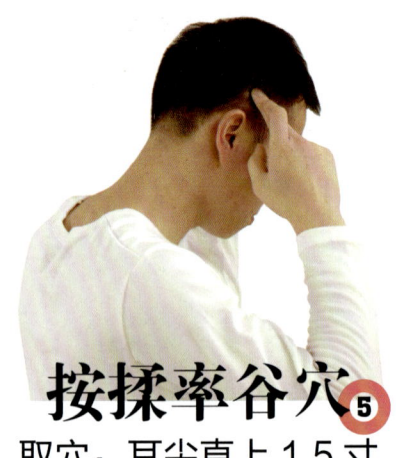

按揉率谷穴 ❺
取穴：耳尖直上1.5寸

方法
用两手中指螺纹面同时按揉100次。

要领
手法用力宜适中，带动皮下组织按揉，使颞部有轻松感，局部有轻度酸痛感。

Press and knead Shuai Gu point
Location
1.5 cun above the tip of the ear.

Manipulation
Press and knead the points with both middle fingers, 100 times.

Key
Press and knead the point together with the soft tissue underneath with medium force, relaxing the temporal area.

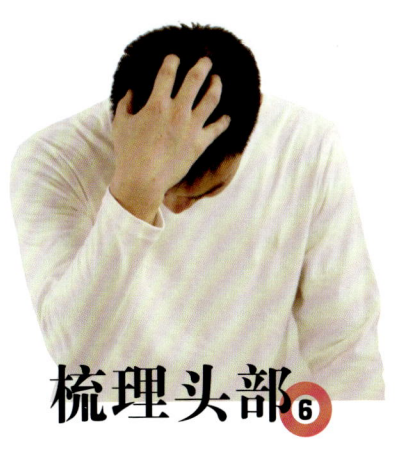

梳理头部 ⑥

方法
用五指螺纹面自前发际向头后部梳理 30 次。

要领
手指螺纹面紧贴头部皮肤，自前向后梳理，手法用力宜适中，使头部有轻松和温热感。

Comb hair

Manipulation

Comb with five fingers from front hairline to the back, 30 times.

Key

Press and knead the point together with the soft tissue underneath with medium force, relaxing the temporal area and making it feel warm.

慢性结肠炎
Chronic Colitis

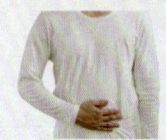

1 抚摩下腹部
Massage lower abdomen

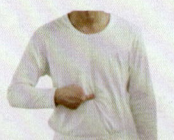

2 按揉中脘穴
Press and knead Zhong Wan point

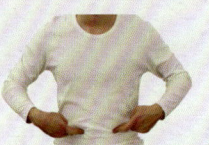

3 按揉天枢穴
Press and knead Tian Shu point

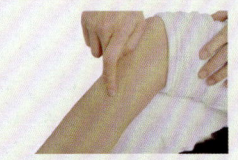

4 按揉足三里穴
Press and knead Zu San Li point

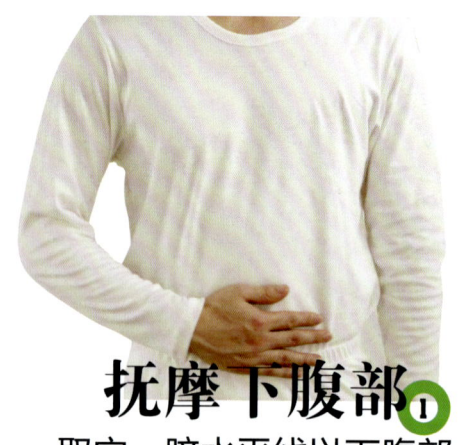

抚摩下腹部 ①
取穴：脐水平线以下腹部

方法
用手掌面在下腹部做逆时针方向抚摩 100 次。

要领
按左下腹→左上腹→右上腹→右下腹→左下腹的顺序进行，手法用力宜轻柔，使腹部有温热感。

Massage lower abdomen
Location
Abdomen below umbilicus.

Manipulation
Stroke anticlockwise 100 times with your palm on lower abdomen.

Key
Stroke with gentle force by following the order of left low → left up → right up → right low → left low on the lower abdomen, making the abdomen feel warm.

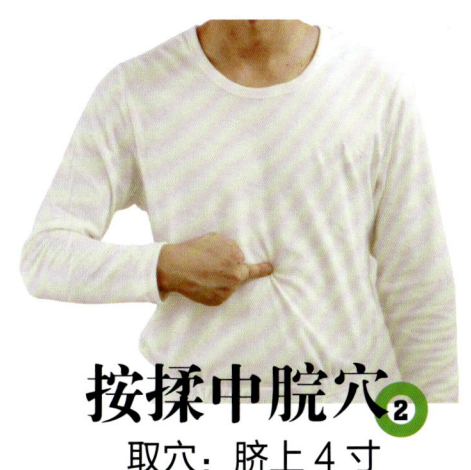

按揉中脘穴 ②
取穴：脐上4寸

方法
用中指螺纹面按揉100次。
要领
手法用力宜适中，使局部有温热感和通气感。

Press and knead Zhong Wan point
Location
4 cun above umbilicus.
Manipulation
Press and knead with middle finger, 100 times.
Key
Use medium force and make the abdomen feel warm.

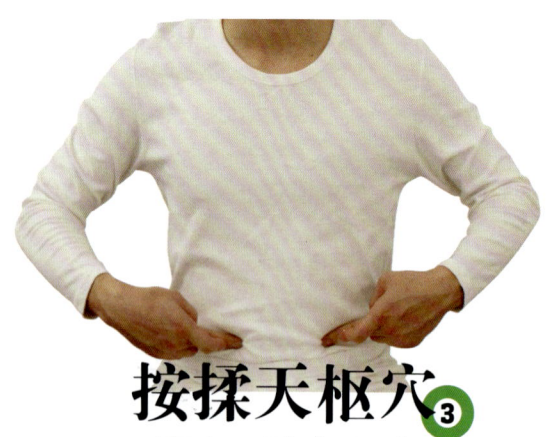

按揉天枢穴 ③
取穴：脐旁 2 寸

方法
用中指螺纹面按揉，左右各 100 次。
要领
双手中指同时按揉，手法用力宜适中，使局部有温热感。

Press and knead Tian Shu point
Location
2 cun lateral to umbilicus.
Manipulation
Press and knead with middle finger, 100 times each side.
Key
Press and knead with both fingers with medium force and make the abdomen feel warm.

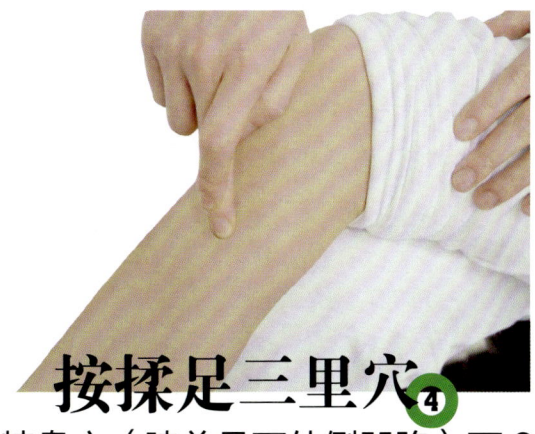

按揉足三里穴 ❹

取穴：犊鼻穴（膝盖骨下外侧凹陷）下3寸，胫骨前嵴（小腿部最突出骨骼处）外一横指

方法
用两手中指指端同时按揉100次。

要领
双膝屈曲，两手中指同时在穴位上按揉，手法用力宜深沉，使局部有酸胀感和温热感。

Press and knead Zu San Li point

Location

3 cun directly below Du Bi point, 1 cun lateral to the anterior border of the tibia.

Manipulation

Press and knead with both middle fingers, 100 times.

Key

Flex the knees and manipulate with deep and strong force to create soreness.

慢性结肠炎

习惯性便秘
Constipation

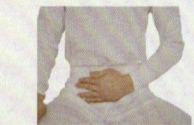

1 抚摩下腹部
Massage lower abdomen

2 按揉中脘穴
Press and knead Zhong Wan point

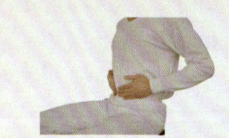

3 按揉大横穴、天枢穴
Press and knead Da Heng & Tian Shu point

4 **按揉支沟穴**
Press and knead Zhi Gou point

5 **按揉足三里穴**
Press and knead Zu San Li point

6 **擦腰部脊柱两侧**
Rub both sides of lumbar spine

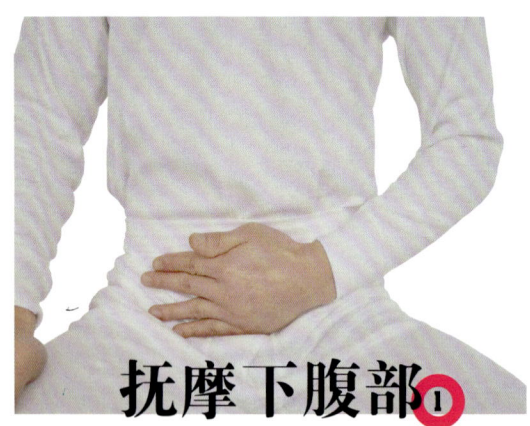

抚摩下腹部 ①
取穴：脐水平线以下腹部

方法
用手掌面在下腹部做顺时针方向抚摩 100 次。

要领
按右下腹→右上腹→左上腹→左下腹→右下腹的顺序进行，手法用力宜轻柔，使腹部有温热感。

Massage lower abdomen
Location
Abdomen below umbilicus.
Manipulation
Stroke clockwise 100 times with your palm on lower abdomen.
Key
Stroke with gentle force by following the order of right low → right up → left up → left low → right low on the lower abdomen, making the abdomen feel warm.

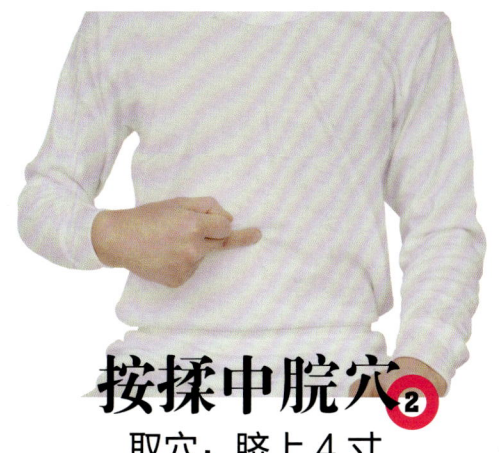

按揉中脘穴 ❷
取穴：脐上 4 寸

方法
用中指螺纹面按揉 100 次。
要领
手法用力宜适中，使局部有温热感和通气感。

Press and knead Zhong Wan point
Location
4 cun above umbilicus.
Manipulation
Press and knead with middle finger, 100 times.
Key
Use medium force and make the abdomen feel warm.

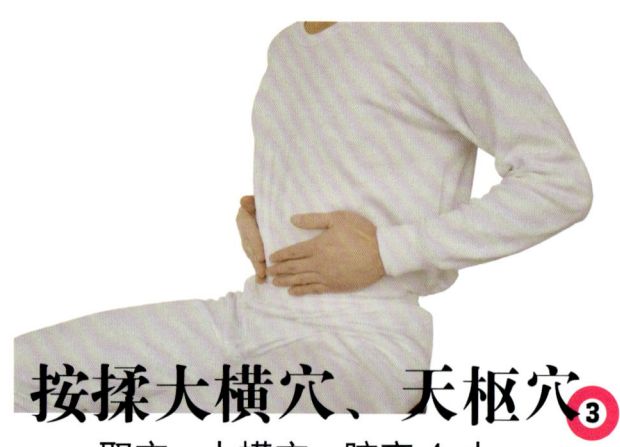

按揉大横穴、天枢穴 ③

取穴：大横穴：脐旁4寸；
天枢穴：脐旁2寸

方法
用手掌顺时针按揉，左右各100次。

要领
两侧穴位均做顺时针方向按揉，
手法用力宜适中，使局部有温热感。

Press and knead Da Heng & Tian Shu point

Location
Da Heng point: 4 cun lateral to umbilicus.
Tian Shu point: 2 cun lateral to umbilicus.

Manipulation
Press and knead clockwise with the palm, 100 times each side.

Key
Press and knead clockwise with medium force
and make the abdomen feel warm.

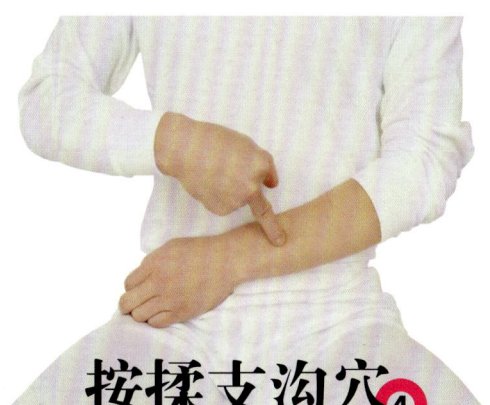

按揉支沟穴 ❹

取穴：腕背横纹上3寸，尺骨与桡骨之间（手臂中间）

方法
用中指螺纹面按揉，左右各100次。

要领
左手按揉右侧穴位，右手按揉左侧穴位，手法用力宜深沉，使局部有酸胀感。

Press and knead Zhi Gou point

Location

3 cun above the dorsal radiocarpal transverse crease, between the ulnar and radius.

Manipulation

Press and knead with middle finger, 100 times each side.

Key

Manipulate with deep and strong force and make the point feel sore.

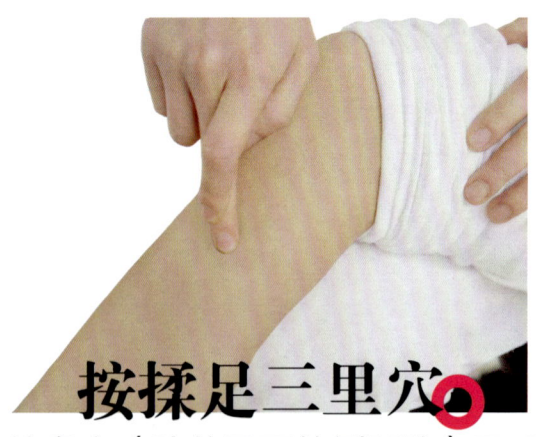

按揉足三里穴

取穴：犊鼻穴（膝盖骨下外侧凹陷）下3寸，胫骨前嵴（小腿部最突出骨骼处）外一横指

方法
用中指指端按揉，左右各100次。

要领
双手中指同时按揉，手法用力宜偏重，使局部有酸胀感和温热感。

Press and knead Zu San Li point
Location
3 cun directly below Du Bi point,
1 cun lateral to the anterior border of the tibia.
Manipulation
Press and knead with middle finger, 100 times each side.
Key
Manipulate with deep and strong force and make the point feel sore and warm.

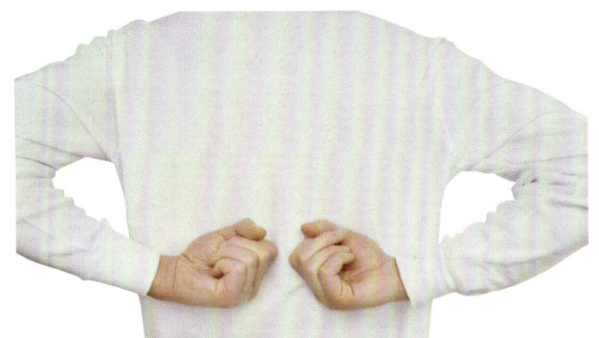

擦腰部脊柱两侧 ❻

取穴：腰部脊柱两侧（脾俞穴至大肠俞穴：第十一胸椎至第四腰椎棘突下，旁开 1.5 寸）

方法
两手握空拳，用拳眼在腰部两侧做上下往返摩擦 50 次。

要领
拳眼紧贴体表，手法用力宜适中，
节奏宜稍快，使局部有明显温热感。

Rub both sides of lumbar spine
Location
Both sides of lumbar spine.
Manipulation
Make a hollow fist and rub both sides of the lumbar spine, 50 times.
Key
The fist touches the body firmly, rub quickly with medium force and make the local area feel warm.

视疲劳
Eye Fatigue

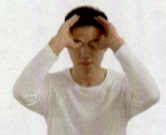

1 推揉睛明穴
Push and knead Jing Ming point

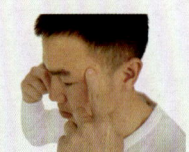

2 按揉太阳穴
Press and knead Tai Yang point

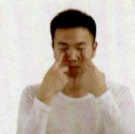

3 按揉承泣穴
Press and knead Cheng Qi point

4 按揉风池穴
Press and knead Feng Chi point

5 熨双眼
Warm both eyes

6 按揉鱼腰穴
Press and knead Yu Yao point

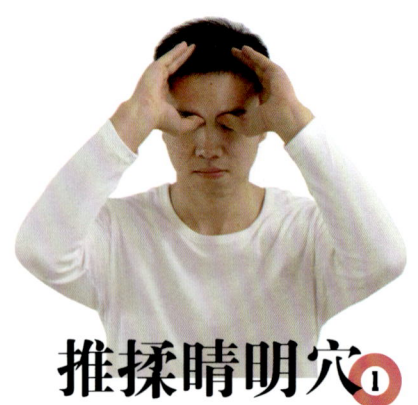

推揉睛明穴 ❶
取穴：目内眦旁 0.1 寸（目内眦角上方凹陷处）

方法

用两手拇指指端向内上同时推揉 100 次。

要领

双手拇指同时向内上方推揉，勿触压眼球，手法用力宜轻柔，使局部有酸胀感。

Push and knead Jing Ming point

Location

0.1 cun above the inner canthus.

Manipulation

Push and knead with both thumbs, 100 times.

Key

Push and knead upwards. Do not touch eyeballs. Use gentle force until it feels sore.

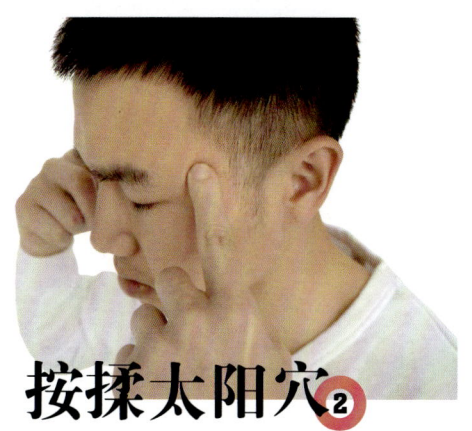

按揉太阳穴 ②
取穴：眉梢与目外眦之间
向后约 1 寸凹陷处

方法
用双手食指螺纹面同时按揉 100 次。
要领
操作时精神要放松，意念集中于太阳穴，手法用力宜轻柔，
带动皮下组织按揉，使局部有舒适感。

Press and knead Tai Yang point
Location
1 cun posterior to the eyebrow and outer canthus.
Manipulation
Press and knead the points with both index fingers, 100 times.
Key
Relax and focus your mind on Tai Yang point. Use gentle force
and knead together with the soft tissue underneath.

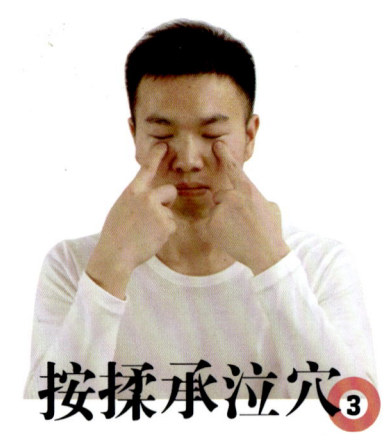

按揉承泣穴 ③
取穴：瞳孔直下，当眶下缘与眼球之间
（眼球正下方，眼眶骨凹陷处）

方法
用两手食指指端同时按揉 100 次。
要领
两指同时按揉，勿触压眼球，
手法用力宜适中，使局部有酸胀感。

Press and knead Cheng Qi point
Location
Directly below the pupil and between the eyeball
and the infraorbital ridge.
Manipulation
Press and knead with both index fingers, 100 times.
Key
Push and knead with both fingers at the same time and do not touch eyeballs. Use gentle force until it feels sore.

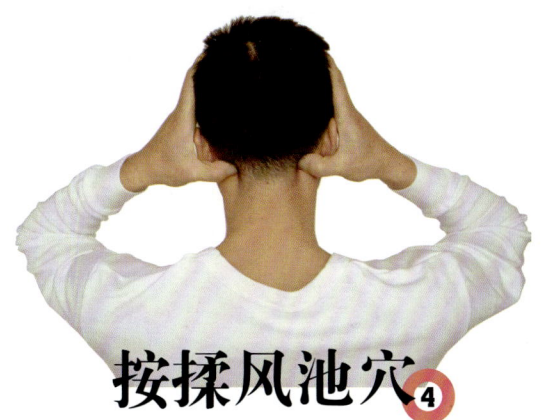

按揉风池穴 ④

取穴：十指自然张开抱头，拇指往上推，在脖子与发际的交界线各有一凹处（风府穴与颞骨乳突之间的凹陷处）

方法
用双手拇指螺纹面同时按揉 100 次。

要领
拇指螺纹面按于风池穴紧贴枕骨上缘，向内上按揉，使颞侧头部有放射样酸胀麻感。

Press and knead Feng Chi point

Location

Hold the back of head with ten fingers upwards, your thumb will find a depression between the upper ends of the sternocleidomastoid and trapezius muscles.

Manipulation

Press and knead the points with both thumbs, 100 times.

Key

Touch the upper edge of occipital bone with the thumb firmly and manipulate upwards, soreness should radiate to the temporal area.

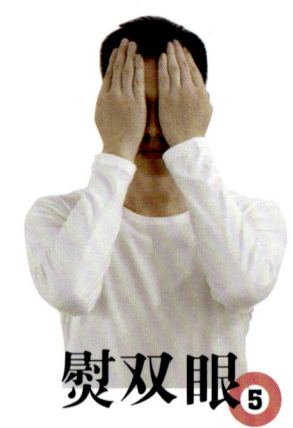

熨双眼 ⑤

方法
双手掌心相对搓热，熨捂双眼，重复操作 5 次。
要领
熨捂时双眼闭合，意念集中于眼睛，使双眼有温热感。

Warm both eyes
Manipulation
Rub both your palms together until they get warm and place them on the eyes, repeat 5 times.
Key
While manipulating, close your eyes and focus your mind on the eyes.

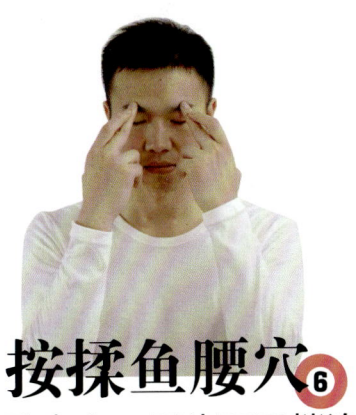

按揉鱼腰穴 ❻
取穴：瞳孔直上，眉头至眉梢连线中点

方法
用双手中指螺纹面同时按揉 100 次。
要领
手法用力宜适中，使局部有酸胀感。

Press and knead Yu Yao point
Location
At midpoint of the eyebrow.
Manipulation
Press and knead the points with both middle fingers, 100 times.
Key
Manipulate the point with medium force.

牙痛
Toothache

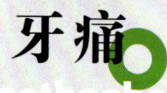

1 按揉下关穴
Press and knead Xia Guan point

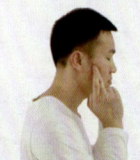

2 按揉颊车穴
Press and knead Jia Che point

按揉痛点
Press and knead tender point

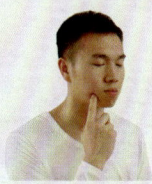

按揉合谷穴
Press and knead He Gu point

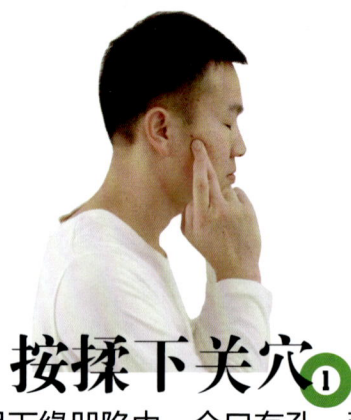

按揉下关穴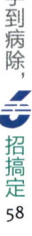

取穴：颧弓下缘凹陷中，合口有孔，张口即闭（闭口，食指、中指并拢，食指贴于耳垂旁，中指指腹处即是）

方法
用中指螺纹面按揉患侧下关穴100次。

要领
按揉患侧穴位，手法用力宜适中，使局部有酸胀感和温热感。

Press and knead Xia Guan point

Location

In the depression below the zygomatic arch. When you close your mouth you can feel it.

Manipulation

Press and knead with middle finger, 100 times.

Key

Press and knead the point with medium force and make it feel warm and sore.

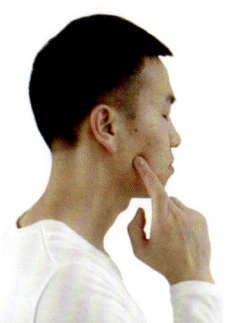

按揉颊车穴 ❷

取穴：下颌角前上方一横指凹陷中，
咀嚼时咬肌隆起最高点（咬紧牙时肌肉突起处）

方法
用食指螺纹面按揉患侧颊车穴100次。

要领
按揉患侧穴位，手法用力宜适中，
使局部有酸胀感和温热麻木感。

Press and knead Jia Che point

Location

1 cun anterosuperior to the mandibular angle.

Manipulation

Press and knead with index finger, 100 times.

Key

Press and knead the point with medium force and make it feel warm and sore.

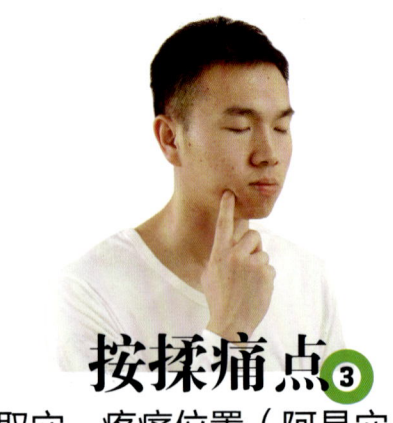

按揉痛点 ③
取穴：疼痛位置（阿是穴）

方法
用食指螺纹面按揉患侧痛点 100 次。
要领
在疼痛明显处按揉，手法用力由轻到重，
使局部有酸胀感或酸痛感。

Press and knead tender point
Location
Tender point.
Manipulation
Press and knead tender point with index finger, 100 times.
Key
Press and knead tender point with medium force and
make it feel warm and sore.

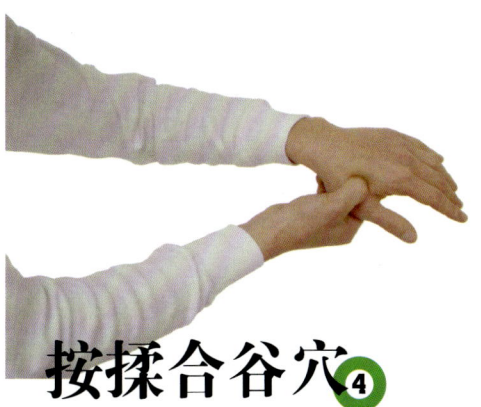

按揉合谷穴 ❹

取穴：虎口，第二掌骨桡侧中点处
（在一手的拇指第一个关节横纹正对另一手的虎口边，拇指屈曲按下，指尖所指处）

方法
用拇指与食指对捏按揉 100 次。

要领
左侧牙痛按揉右侧，右侧牙痛按揉左侧。
手法用力宜深沉，使局部有明显酸胀感或酸痛感。

Press and knead He Gu point

Location

In the middle of the depression radial to the 2nd metacarpal bone, back of the hand. Cross your palms and press the point where the thumb touches.

Manipulation

Press and knead with thumb and index finger, 100 times.

Key

Use strong manipulation and make the point feel sore.

颈椎病
Neck Pain

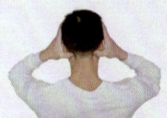

1 按揉风池穴
Press and knead Feng Chi point

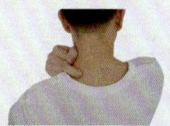

2 按揉颈根穴
Press and knead Jing Gen point

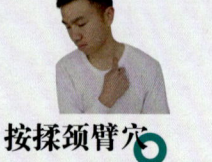

3 按揉颈臂穴
Press and knead Jing Bi point

4 提拿颈旁线
Lift and grasp the neck muscle

5 扳颈后伸法
Pull and extend neck backwards

6 摩擦颈项法
Rub the neck

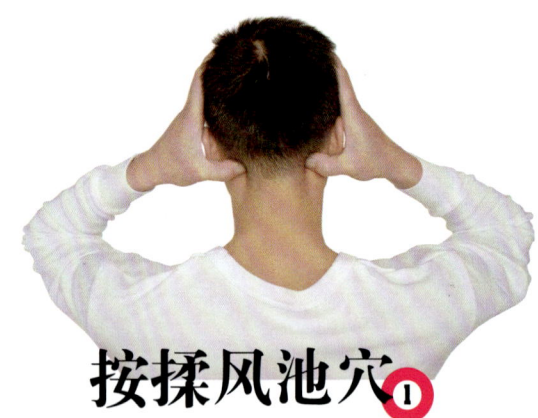

按揉风池穴 ❶

取穴：十指自然张开抱头，拇指往上推，在脖子与发际的交界线各有一凹处（风府穴与颞骨乳突之间的凹陷处）

方法
用双手拇指螺纹面同时按揉 100 次。

要领
拇指螺纹面按于风池穴紧贴枕骨上缘按揉，
使局部有明显酸胀感。

Press and knead Feng Chi point
Location
Hold the back of head with ten fingers upwards,
your thumb will find a depression between the upper ends of the sternocleidomastoid and trapezius muscles.

Manipulation
Press and knead the points with both thumbs, 100 times.

Key
You will feel sore while pressing and kneading the point.

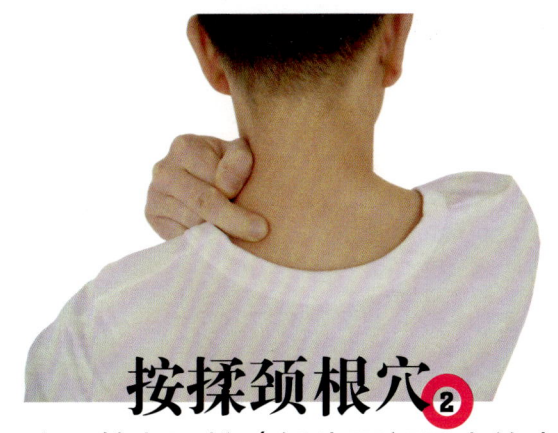

按揉颈根穴 ❷
取穴：第七颈椎（低头颈部最高的点）
下方凹陷处旁开 1.5 寸

方法
用中指指端按揉，左右各 100 次。

要领
左手按揉右侧穴位，右手按揉左侧穴位，
手法用力宜深沉，使局部有酸胀感。

Press and knead Jing Gen point
Location
1.5 cun lateral to the depression below C7
(the highest point on the neck when looking downwards).

Manipulation
Knead with middle finger, 100 times each side.

Key
Press and knead the point with deep and strong force
until you feel sore.

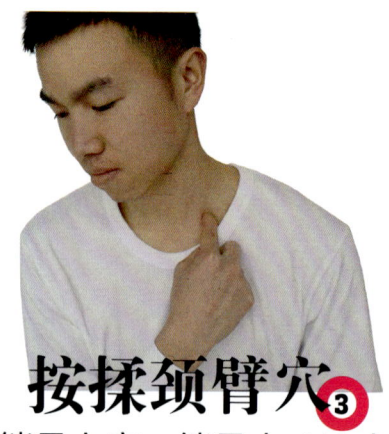

按揉颈臂穴 ❸
取穴：锁骨上窝，锁骨内 1/4 上 1 寸

方法
用食指螺纹面按揉，左右各 100 次。
要领
用左手按揉右侧穴位，右手按揉左侧穴位，
手法用力宜适中，使局部有酸胀感。

Press and knead Jing Bi point
Location
1 cun in supraclavicular fossae, inner 1/4 of collarbone.
Manipulation
Press and knead with index finger, 100 times each side.
Key
Press and knead the point with medium force until you feel sore.

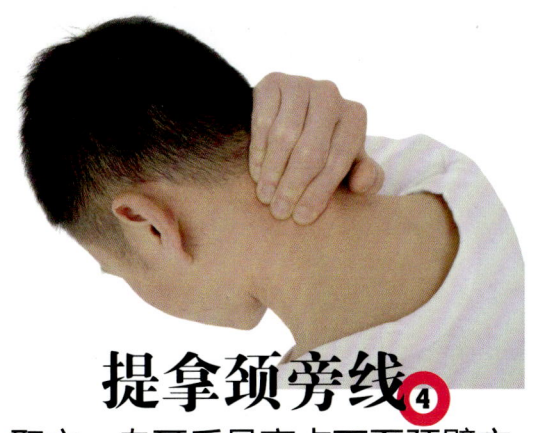

提拿颈旁线 ❹
取穴：自耳后最高点下至颈臂穴

方法
用四指（除拇指外）与掌根部相对用力提拿颈项肌肉，重复操作 9 次。

要领
手法用力宜偏重，捏拿要紧实，提起要缓慢，放开要舒展，使局部有明显温热舒适感。

Lift and grasp the neck muscle
Location
From the highest point behind ear to Jing Bi point.
Manipulation
Lift and grasp muscle with four fingers (except thumb) and the root of the palm, repeat 9 times.
Key
The force should be strong and solid, slowly lifting and relaxing totally, until a warm feeling rises to the local area.

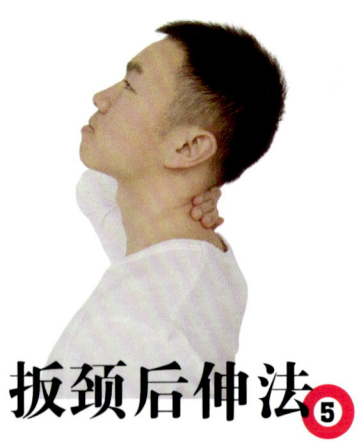

扳颈后伸法 ❺

方法
用四指（除拇指外）按于颈后部，头向后仰，
手向前拉，重复操作 9 次。

要领
手指按压要紧实，头部后仰与手向前拉要同步，形成对抗牵引，
动作要缓慢，不可用蛮力，使颈项有明显舒展感。

Pull and extend neck backwards
Manipulation
Put four fingers (except thumb) on the neck, pull the head back and push your hand forward, repeat for 9 times.

Key
Four fingers should hold tightly when pulling and extending.
It creates a counteraction which should be slow so the neck feels an obvious extension.

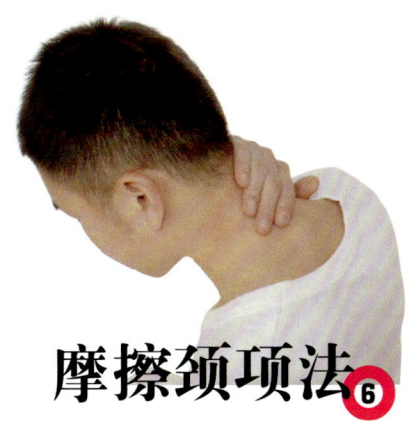

摩擦颈项法 ❻

方法
手掌置于颈后部,左右往返摩擦颈项部,重复操作9次。

要领
手掌紧贴颈项部,摩擦距离宜长,摩擦频率宜缓慢,使局部有明显温热感。

Rub the neck
Manipulation
Put your palm on the neck, rub the neck, 9 times.
Key
Rub as long strokes as possible with slow frequency to bring a warm feeling to the local area.

腰肌劳损
Lumbar Strain

1 按揉阿是穴
Press and knead tender point

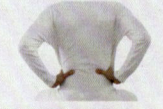

2 按揉委中穴
Press and knead Wei Zhong point

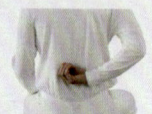

3 叩腰法
Tap lumbar

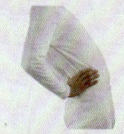

4 叉腰屈伸法
Flex and stretch lumbar area

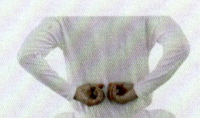

5 擦膀胱经腰段
Rub bladder channel in lumbar region

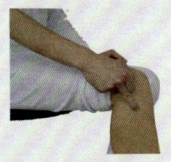

6 按揉阳陵泉穴
Press and knead Yang Ling Quan point

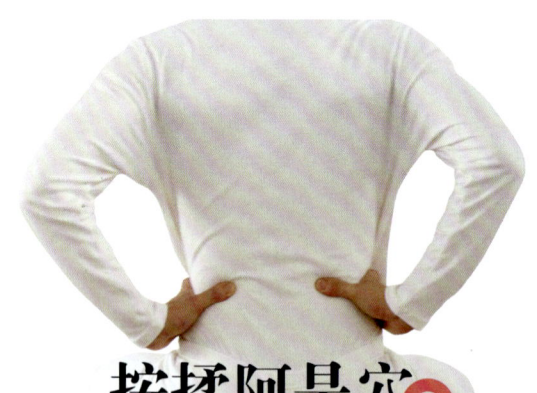

按揉阿是穴 ①
取穴：疼痛位置（阿是穴）

方法
用拇指螺纹面按揉 100 次。
要领
手法用力宜适中，使局部有明显酸胀感或温热感。

Press and knead tender point
Location
Tender point.
Manipulation
Press and knead tender point with thumb, 100 times.
Key
Press and knead tender point with medium force and make it feel warm and sore.

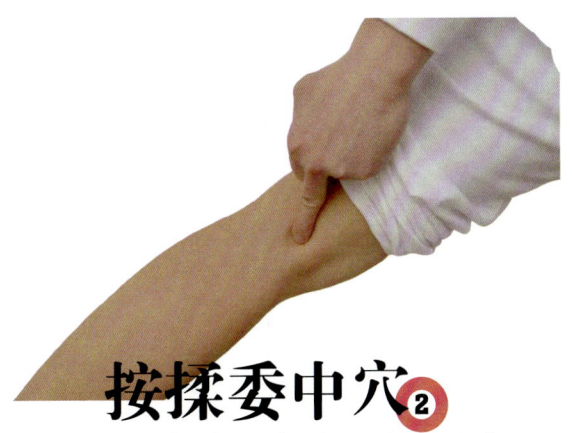

按揉委中穴 ❷
取穴：腘横纹正中（腘窝中央）

方法
用两手中指指端同时按揉 100 次。
要领
双膝屈曲，两手中指勾揉委中穴，手法用力宜深沉，使局部有明显酸胀感。

Press and knead Wei Zhong point
Location
At the midpoint of the transverse crease of the popliteal fossa.
Manipulation
Press and knead the points with both middle fingers, 100 times.
Key
Manipulate the points with strong force while flexing the knees.

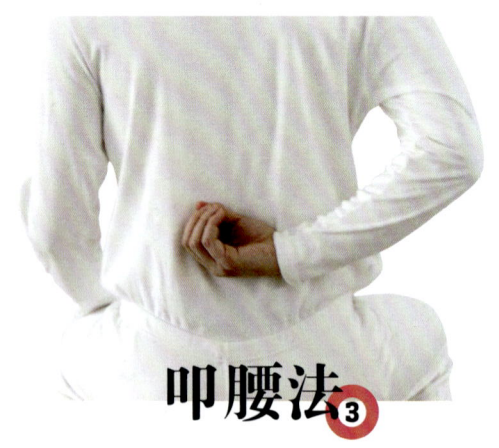

叩腰法 ③

方法
手握空拳,用拳眼叩击腰部 30 次。

要领
用拳眼叩击腰部两侧肌肉,左右手一起一落叩击,
动作要稳实连贯,使腰部有震动感。

Tap lumbar
Manipulation
Tap the lumbar area, 30 times with a hollow fist.
Key
Tap the muscle area with a hollow fist to relax the lumbar region.

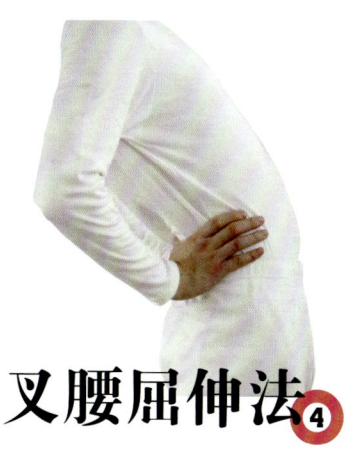

叉腰屈伸法 ❹

方法
双手叉腰，做腰部屈伸活动 30 次。
要领
屈曲动作宜缓慢，后伸动作要伸至最大限度，
并持续片刻，使腰部有舒适感。

Flex and stretch lumbar area
Manipulation
Put your hands on lumbar region, then
flex and extend from the waist, 30 times.
Key
Move slowly and hold when reaching the pain threshold.

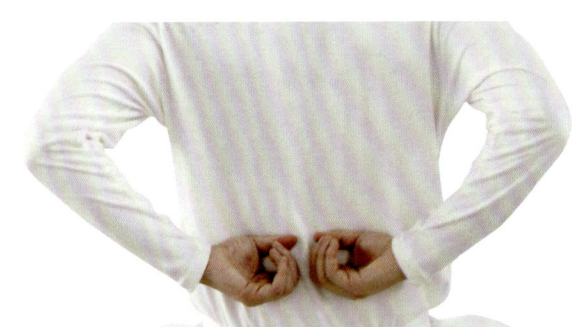

擦膀胱经腰段 ⑤
取穴：脊柱腰段两侧
（脊柱中线旁开，第一侧线 1.5 寸，第二侧线 3 寸）

方法
两手握空拳，用拳眼在腰部两侧膀胱经
做上下往返摩擦 50 次。

要领
拳眼紧贴体表，手法用力宜适中，
节奏宜稍快，使局部有明显温热感。

Rub bladder channel in lumbar region
Location
Both sides of the lumbar spine.
Manipulation
Make a hollow fist and rub both sides of the lumbar spine, 50 times.
Key
The fist firmly touches the body. Rub until it feels warm.

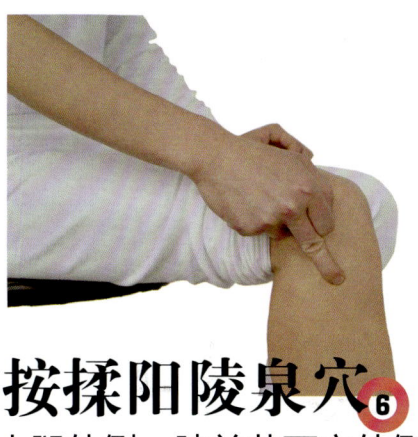

按揉阳陵泉穴 ❻

取穴：小腿外侧，膝关节下方外侧高点（腓骨小头）前下方1寸的凹陷处

方法
用两手中指指端同时按揉100次。

要领
双膝屈曲，两手中指勾揉委中穴，手法用力宜深沉，使局部有明显酸胀感。

Press and knead Yang Ling Quan point

Location

In the depression anterior and inferior to the head of the fibula.

Manipulation

Press and knead the points with both middle fingers, 100 times.

Key

Kneading closely to the head of the fibula will enhance the soreness sensation. The force should be deep and strong.

肩关节周围炎
Shoulder Pain (Frozen Shoulder)

1 揉摩患肩
Knead and rub shoulder

2 按揉肩髃穴
Press and knead Jian Yu point

3 按揉肩贞穴
Press and knead Jian Zhen point

4 托肘运肩
Rotate the shoulder

5 体后拉手
Hold hands behind body

6 压肩摸高
Raise the shoulder

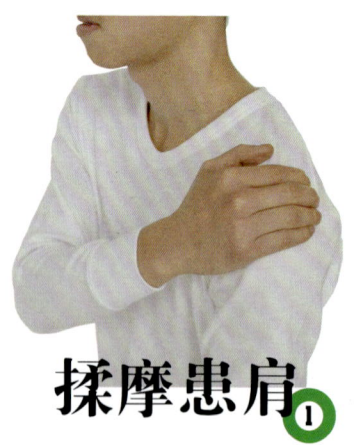

揉摩患肩

方法
用健侧手掌按于患肩部揉摩 100 次。

要领
整个手掌均紧贴皮肤,手法用力宜适中,揉摩范围宜大,以深部透热为佳。

Knead and rub shoulder
Manipulation
Knead and rub painful shoulder with your palm, 100 times.
Key
The whole palm should closely touch the skin and work with medium strength, until the joint feels warm.

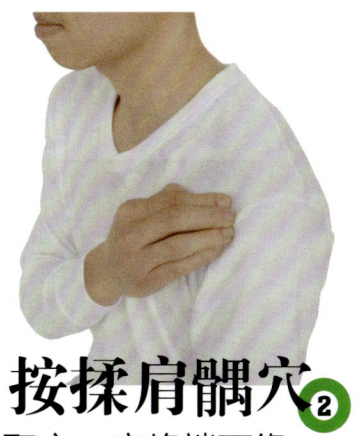

按揉肩髃穴 ❷
取穴：肩峰端下缘，手臂平举时肩前凹陷中

方法
用健侧手的食指、中指、无名指三指指端按揉 100 次。
要领
以肩髃穴为中心进行按揉，手法用力宜适中，使局部有明显酸胀感或酸痛感。

Press and knead Jian Yu point
Location
When arm is fully abducted, a depression will be found at the anterior border of the shoulder joint, where the point is.
Manipulation
Press and knead with index, middle and ring fingers, 100 times.
Key
Manipulate with medium force until it feels sore.

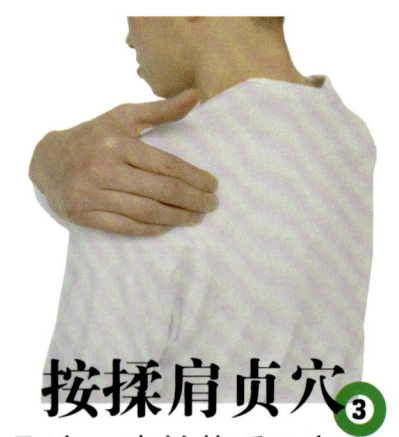

按揉肩贞穴 ❸
取穴：肩关节后下方，
臂内收时，腋后纹头上1寸

方法
用健侧手的食指、中指、无名指三指指端按揉100次。
要领
以肩贞穴为中心进行按揉，手法用力宜适中，
使局部有明显酸胀感或酸痛感。

Press and knead Jian Zhen point
Location
1 cun directly above the posterior end of the axillary fold when the arm is adducted.
Manipulation
Press and knead with index, middle and ring fingers, 100 times.
Key
Manipulate with medium force until the shoulder feels sore.

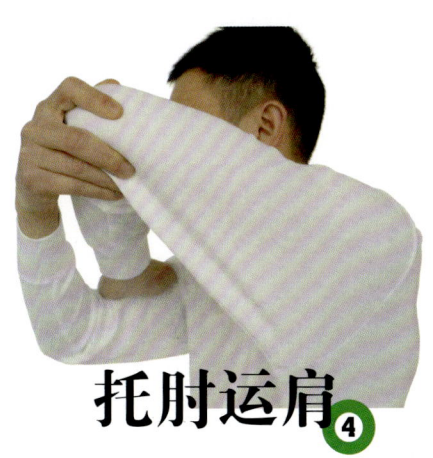

托肘运肩 ④

方法
用健侧手掌托住患肢肘部,做向前、向后运肩各9次。

要领
向前运肩,做肘部向上→向后→向下→向前→向上顺序运肩;
向后运肩,做肘部向下→向后→向上→向前→向下顺序运肩。

Rotate the shoulder

Manipulation
Bend and hold the elbow with your palm, then rotate the shoulder forward and backward, 9 times.

Key
When rotating forwards, the elbow goes upwards → backwards → downwards → forwards → upwards. When rotating backwards, the elbow goes downwards → backwards → upwards → forwards → downwards.

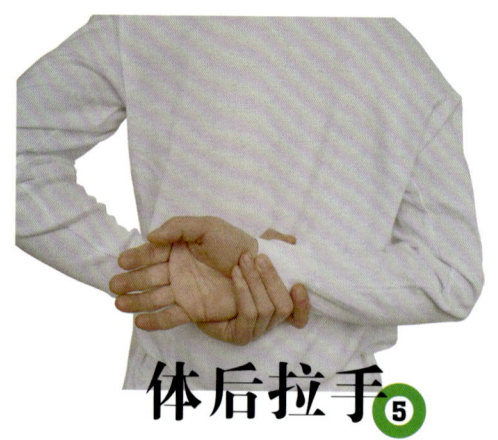

体后拉手 ⑤

方法
用健侧手从背后握住患肢手腕,
做向健侧拉手并向上抬举患肢,重复操作 9 次。

要领
先将患肢向健侧拉,待有一定的紧张感,
再将患肢手腕向上抬举,抬至最大高度时停顿片刻,再放下。

Hold hands behind body

Manipulation
Hold the wrist behind your back, then
pull and lift the hand to the healthy side, repeat 9 times.

Key
Pull the unwell side to the healthy side until pain limits,
then pull the wrist upwards until limited.

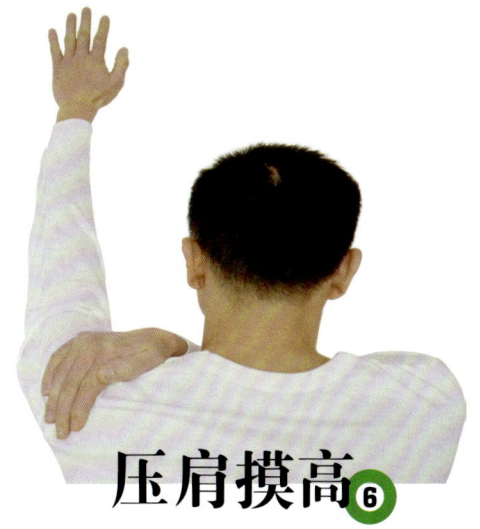

压肩摸高 ❻

方法
面墙而立,患肢上举扶墙摸高,
用健侧手掌按压患肩,重复操作9次。

要领
患肢手指尽可能摸到最高限度时按压患肩,
停顿片刻,再按压患肩,手法要稳实,以能忍受为限。

Raise the shoulder
Manipulation
Face a wall and raise the shoulder as high as possible, then press the shoulder down with your palm, repeat 9 times.

Key
Reach the fingers of unwell side as high as possible and hold for a moment, until pain limited.

增生性膝关节炎
Knee Osteoarthritis

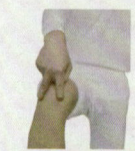

1 按揉膝眼
Press and knead Xi Yan (knee-eyes) point

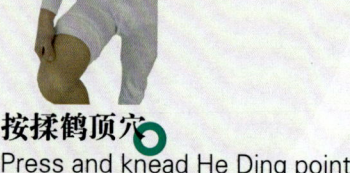

2 按揉鹤顶穴
Press and knead He Ding point

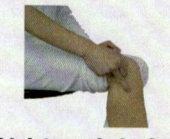

3 按揉阳陵泉穴
Press and knead Yang Ling Quan point

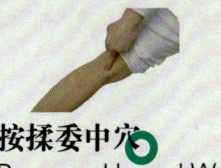

4 按揉委中穴
Press and knead Wei Zhong point

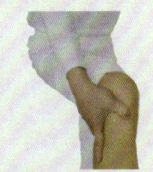

5 按揉髌韧带
Press and knead patellar ligament

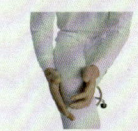

6 按揉膝关节两侧
Press and knead knee joint

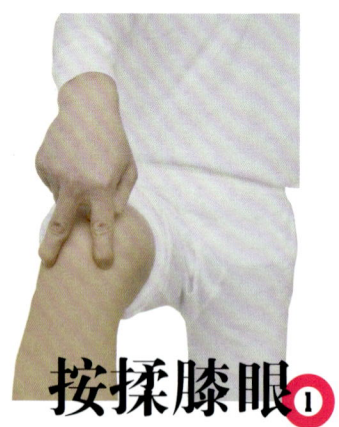

按揉膝眼 ①
取穴：髌骨（膝盖骨）下髌韧带两侧凹陷处

方法
用食指、中指指端同时按揉两侧膝眼 100 次。

要领
双膝屈曲，两指分别在髌韧带两侧的凹陷处进行按揉，手法用力宜适中，使局部有酸胀感。

Press and knead Xi Yan (knee-eyes) point
Location
In the lateral depressions of the patellar ligament.
Manipulation
Press and knead the points with index and middle fingers, 100 times.
Key
Manipulate when knees are flexed and work with medium force.

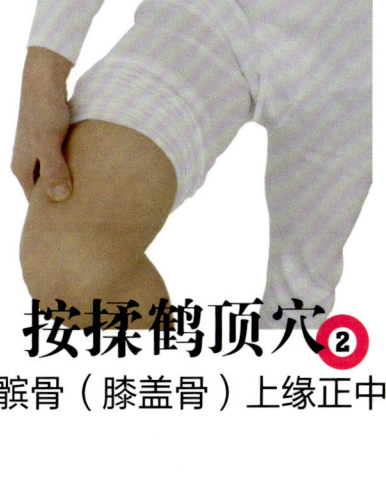

按揉鹤顶穴 ❷
取穴：髌骨（膝盖骨）上缘正中凹陷处

方法
用两手拇指螺纹面同时按揉 100 次。
要领
双膝屈曲，拇指分别在髌骨上缘凹陷处进行按揉，手法用力宜适中，使局部有酸胀感。

Press and knead He Ding point
Location
In the depression on the midpoint of the upper border of patella.
Manipulation
Press and knead the points with both thumbs, 100 times.
Key
Manipulate the point when knees are flexed and work with medium force.

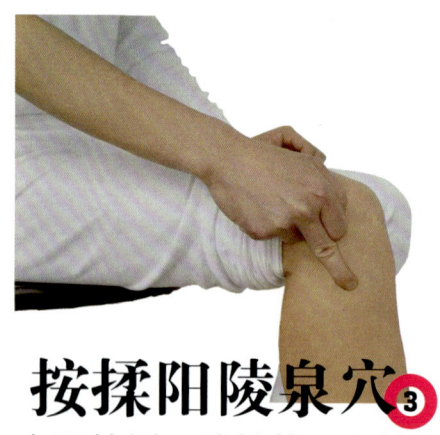

按揉阳陵泉穴 ❸

取穴：小腿外侧，膝关节下方外侧高点（腓骨小头）前下方 1 寸的凹陷处

方法
用两手中指指端同时按揉 100 次。

要领
指端贴近腓骨小头缘按揉可增强感应，手法用力宜深沉偏重，使局部有酸胀感。

Press and knead Yang Ling Quan point
Location
In the depression anterior and inferior to the head of the fibula.
Manipulation
Press and knead the points with both middle fingers, 100 times.
Key
Kneading closely to the head of the fibula will enhance the soreness sensation. The force should be deep and strong.

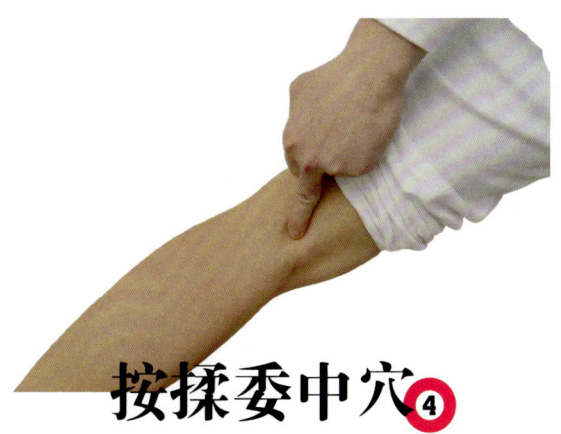

按揉委中穴 ④
取穴：腘横纹正中（腘窝中央）

方法
用两手中指指端同时按揉 100 次。

要领
双膝屈曲，两手中指勾揉委中穴，
手法用力宜偏重，使局部有明显酸胀感。

Press and knead Wei Zhong point
Location
At the midpoint of the transverse crease of the popliteal fossa.
Manipulation
Press and knead the points with both middle fingers, 100 times.
Key
Manipulate the points while bending the knees with strong force.

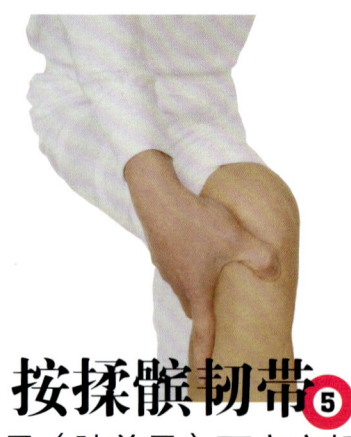

按揉髌韧带 ❺
取穴：髌骨（膝盖骨）下方突起的韧带

方法

用拇指螺纹面分别按揉两侧髌韧带，左右各 100 次。

要领

双膝屈曲，两拇指在髌韧带处进行按揉，
手法用力宜适中，使局部有轻度酸胀感。

Press and knead patellar ligament
Location

The ligament below patella.

Manipulation

Press and knead the point with thumb, 100 times each side.

Key

Manipulate the point when the knees are flexed and
work with medium force.

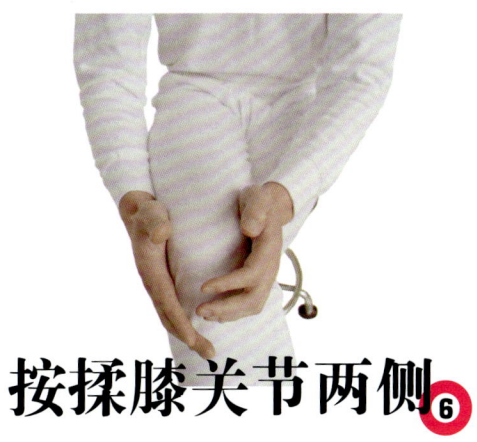

按揉膝关节两侧 ❻

方法
用两手掌根部按揉膝关节内侧和外侧，各 100 次。
要领
手掌根部着力，按揉外侧时两手同时进行；按揉内侧时，
左手按揉右侧，右手按揉左侧。手法用力宜适中，
使局部有明显温热感。

Press and knead knee joint
Manipulation
Press and knead with both palms, 100 times.
Key
Manipulate with the base of the palm with medium force and make the knee joint feel warm.

跟痛症
Heel Pain Syndrome

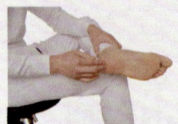

1. 按摩跟底部
Rub the bottom of the heel

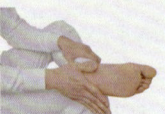

2. 按揉跟底压痛点
Press and knead tender points of heel

3. 掌摩跟底压痛点
Rub the most tender point of the heel

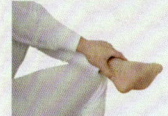

4. 按揉跟腱
Press and knead achilles tendon

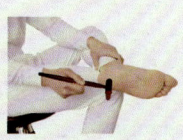

5. 擦跟底部
Rub the bottom of the foot

6. 敲击法
Tapping

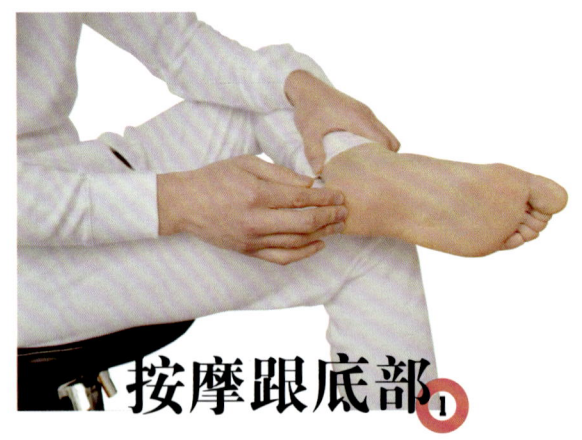

按摩跟底部

方法
用食指、中指、无名指按揉 100 次。

要领
患足搁于健侧膝关节上，用手指螺纹面在跟底部按摩，手法用力宜轻柔。

Rub the bottom of the heel

Manipulation

Press and knead with index, middle and ring fingers, 100 times.

Key

Put the painful heel on your healthy knee joint and knead gently with your fingers.

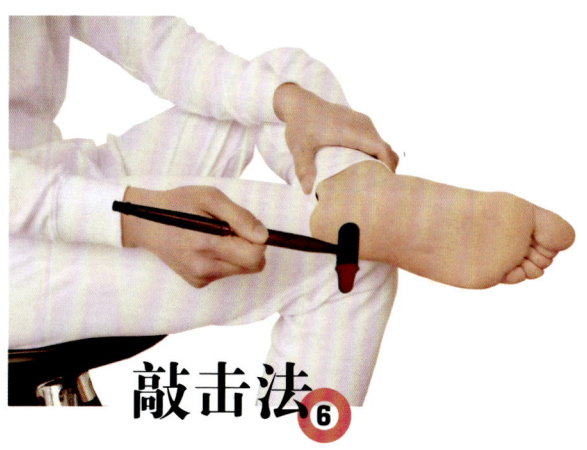

敲击法 ❻

方法
敲击骨刺疼痛部位 1~2 分钟。

要领
一手持敲击物对准患侧足跟压痛点敲击，手腕用力，快速而有节奏，以能忍受为限。

Tapping
Manipulation
Tap the tender area, 1~2 minutes.
Key
Tap the tender area with a solid stuff rapidly and randomly, with sustained force.

慢性鼻炎
Chronic Rhinitis

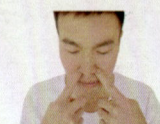

1 按揉迎香穴
Press and knead Ying Xiang point

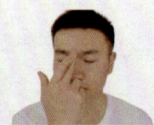

2 按揉印堂穴
Press and knead Yin Tang point

3 按揉风池穴
Press and knead Feng Chi point

4 摩擦鼻旁
Rub nosewing

5 按揉合谷穴
Press and knead He Gu point

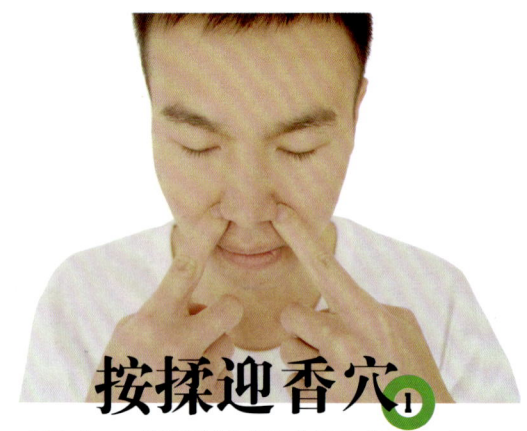

按揉迎香穴
取穴：鼻翼外缘旁开 0.5 寸

方法

用两手食指螺纹面同时按揉 100 次。

要领

两侧穴位同时按揉，手法用力宜适中，频率宜稍快，使局部有酸胀感。

Press and knead Ying Xiang point

Location

0.5 cun lateral to the nosewing under the cheekbone.

Manipulation

Press and knead the points with both index fingers, 100 times.

Key

Manipulate both sides at the same time with medium force and quick frequency, causing soreness in the local area.

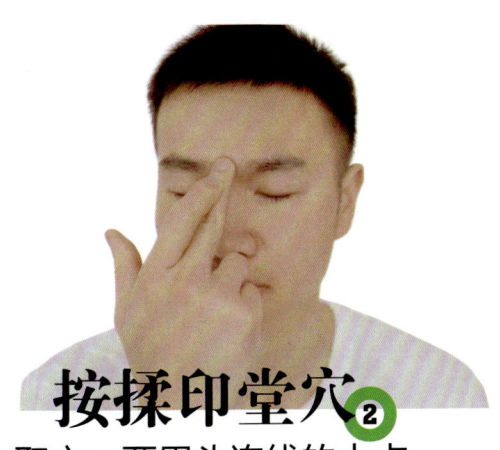

按揉印堂穴 ❷
取穴：两眉头连线的中点

方法

用中指螺纹面按揉 100 次。

要领

手法用力宜轻柔，带动皮下组织按揉。

Press and knead Yin Tang point

Location

At the midpoint of the connecting line between the ends of the two eyebrows.

Manipulation

Press and knead the point with middle finger, 100 times.

Key

Press and knead the point together with the soft tissue underneath with gentle force.

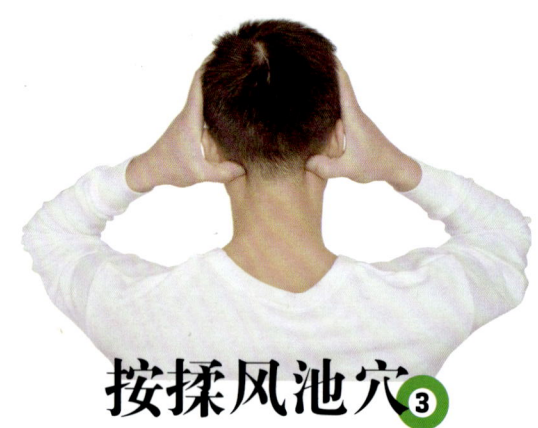

按揉风池穴 ❸

取穴：十指自然张开抱头，拇指往上推，在脖子与发际的交界线各有一凹处（风府穴与颞骨乳突之间的凹陷处）

方法
用双手拇指螺纹面同时按揉 100 次。

要领
拇指螺纹面按于风池穴紧贴枕骨上缘按揉，使局部有酸胀麻感。

Press and knead Feng Chi point

Location

Hold the back of head with ten fingers upwards, your thumb will find a depression between the upper ends of the sternocleidomastoid and trapezius muscles.

Manipulation

Press and knead the points with both thumbs, 100 times.

Key

You will feel sore while pressing and kneading the point.

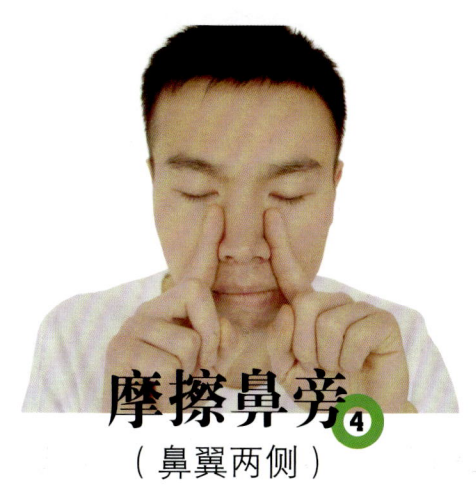

摩擦鼻旁 ④
（鼻翼两侧）

方法
用两手食指在鼻翼两旁上下摩擦 50 次。
要领
两手同时摩擦，手法用力宜轻柔。

Rub nosewing
Manipulation
Rub nosewing 50 times with both index fingers.
Key
Rub with both hands at the same time with gentle force.

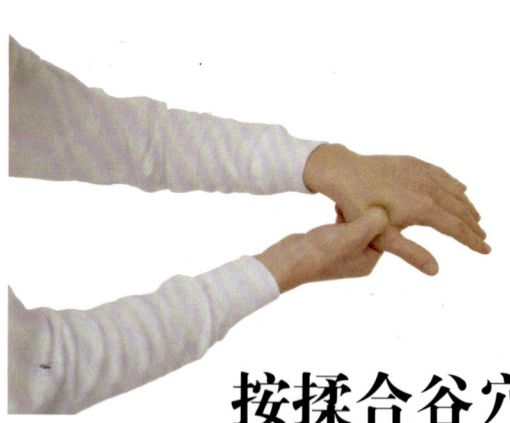

按揉合谷穴 ❺

取穴：虎口，第二掌骨桡侧中点处
（在一手的拇指第一个关节横纹正对另一手的虎口边，
拇指屈曲按下，指尖所指处）

方法
用拇指与食指对捏按揉 100 次。

要领
手法用力宜偏重，使局部有明显酸胀感或酸痛感。

Press and knead He Gu point

Location

In the middle of the depression radial to the 2nd metacarpal bone, back of the hand. Cross your palms and press the point where the thumb touches.

Manipulation

Press and knead with thumb and index finger, 100 times.

Key

Use strong manipulation and cause soreness in the local area.